Painless Procedures

Exploring Minimally Invasive Anesthesia And Sedation Methods

Zane Abernathy

Table of Contents

1 Introduction to Minimally Invasive Techniques

Minimally invasive techniques represent a significant advancement in medical procedures, offering numerous benefits over traditional methods. Their core principle lies in accessing the target area through smaller incisions, utilizing specialized instruments and imaging technology for precision. This approach significantly reduces trauma to surrounding tissues, leading to less postoperative pain and faster healing times. The reduced invasiveness translates to shorter hospital stays, quicker return to normal activities, and a lower risk of complications like infection. This shift towards minimally invasive procedures reflects a broader movement within healthcare towards less invasive and more patient-centered approaches.

The transition to minimally invasive techniques also impacts anesthesia and sedation. Traditional general anesthesia, often associated with prolonged recovery and potential side effects, can be replaced or augmented by less potent, more targeted anesthetic strategies. This might involve regional anesthesia, focusing the anesthetic effect on a specific area, or conscious sedation, allowing the patient to maintain a degree of responsiveness. The selection of the anesthetic technique is highly individualized, based on the specific procedure, patient characteristics, and the preference of both the patient and the anesthesiologist. Thorough patient assessment and clear communication are crucial to make informed decisions.

Understanding the advantages of minimally invasive anesthesia is crucial for any medical professional. These benefits extend beyond the patient's immediate experience. For healthcare systems, these techniques frequently mean lower costs associated with shorter hospital stays and fewer complications needing additional treatment. This cost-effectiveness doesn't compromise patient safety; in fact, many studies have demonstrated reduced infection rates and fewer post-operative complications compared to traditional, more invasive procedures. Such improvements directly contribute to better patient outcomes and increased efficiency within healthcare systems. The reduction in post-operative pain, in particular, leads to improved patient satisfaction and potentially reduces the need for strong analgesics, also impacting patient health outcomes positively.

Furthermore, minimally invasive approaches allow for greater procedural precision. Smaller incisions mean less tissue damage, minimizing scarring and improving cosmetic results. The use of advanced imaging technologies, such as ultrasound or endoscopy, provides real-time visualization, guiding the surgeon with accuracy and enhancing the effectiveness of the procedure. This heightened precision reduces the likelihood of unintentional damage to nearby organs or structures, significantly improving patient safety. The combination of minimal invasiveness and enhanced precision ultimately enhances the overall success rate of many surgical procedures. This underscores the importance of the proper training and expertise of surgical teams using these advanced techniques.

However, it is important to note that minimally invasive techniques are not without their own set of challenges. Specialized training and expertise are necessary for both the surgeons and the anesthesia providers. The use of sophisticated instruments and imaging technology requires a higher level of skill and knowledge. The learning curve can be steep, but the benefits for patients are clear. Investment in advanced equipment and ongoing professional development are therefore essential elements for institutions embracing this approach. The transition to minimally invasive techniques is not merely about adopting new technologies, it demands a holistic change in surgical and anesthesia practices.

Finally, the choice of a minimally invasive technique should always involve shared decision-making with the patient. It's not simply a matter of the surgeon deciding the best approach; the patient's preferences, medical history, and the potential risks and benefits of each option must be thoroughly discussed. Informed consent is paramount, ensuring that the patient has a complete understanding of the procedure, its implications, and the potential alternatives. This transparent and collaborative approach highlights the ethical dimension of adopting minimally invasive approaches, making sure patient autonomy and well-being are prioritized throughout the process. This shared decision-making model underpins the successful and safe implementation of minimally invasive techniques, placing the patient at the heart of the process.

1.1 Defining Minimally Invasive Anesthesia

Minimally invasive anesthesia prioritizes patient comfort and rapid recovery. It's a paradigm shift from traditional general anesthesia, aiming to reduce the invasiveness of the procedure and the associated risks. We're talking about techniques that minimize tissue trauma, leading to less postoperative pain, shorter hospital stays, and a quicker return to normal activities. This approach isn't simply about using smaller incisions; it encompasses a holistic strategy involving careful patient selection, precise anesthetic delivery, and meticulous postoperative care.

Unlike general anesthesia, which renders the patient completely unconscious, minimally invasive approaches often involve techniques that maintain varying levels of consciousness and awareness. This can range from conscious sedation, where the patient can respond to verbal commands, to regional anesthesia, which numbs a specific area of the body. This controlled approach allows for better patient interaction and reduces the risk of complications associated with deep general anesthesia.

The selection of the most appropriate technique depends heavily on the specifics of the surgical procedure itself. A short, minor outpatient procedure might benefit from local infiltration with a topical anesthetic cream. Conversely, a more extensive procedure might necessitate a combined approach using regional anesthesia supplemented by conscious sedation. Therefore, a thorough understanding of the procedural requirements is paramount before selecting an appropriate anesthetic technique.

The core principle behind minimally invasive anesthesia involves optimizing the balance between providing adequate analgesia and minimizing the side effects. This delicate balance requires a skilled anesthetist who can assess the individual patient's needs and tailor the anesthetic plan accordingly. Factors like patient age, medical history, and the nature of the surgery will guide the choice of anesthetic agents and the monitoring strategies implemented.

Effective monitoring is crucial throughout the procedure. Continuous monitoring of vital signs, such as heart rate, blood pressure, and oxygen saturation, is essential for ensuring patient safety. Early detection and management of any potential complications, such as hypotension or respiratory depression, are key to a successful outcome. This continuous vigilance allows for prompt intervention should any issues arise, mitigating potential risks.

Patient education plays a pivotal role in minimally invasive anesthesia. A well-informed patient understands the procedure, the potential benefits and risks, and their role in the process. This fosters trust and collaboration, enhancing the overall experience and leading to a smoother and more successful outcome. Open communication is essential for addressing any questions or concerns.

Beyond the immediate procedural benefits, minimally invasive anesthesia often translates to better long-term patient outcomes. Reduced post-operative pain and discomfort means less reliance on opioid analgesics, consequently lowering the risk of opioid-related side effects, such as addiction or respiratory complications. Ultimately, the goal is not just to anesthetize the patient, but to ensure their comfort, safety, and a swift and smooth recovery. This approach reflects a contemporary focus on enhanced patient experience and superior outcomes.

The ongoing evolution of anesthetic techniques and technological advancements further supports the adoption of minimally invasive methods. New anesthetic agents, more refined delivery systems, and advanced monitoring technologies continually refine the precision and safety of these approaches. This ongoing development holds the promise of even less invasive and more effective anesthetic management in the future. The field is continuously striving for optimization, leading to the improved patient outcomes.

The selection of an anesthetic technique is not solely dictated by procedural considerations but must also incorporate an ethical dimension. The patient's autonomy and right to informed consent are paramount. Open communication and shared decision-making ensure the patient feels involved and confident in the chosen approach, further enhancing the overall experience. Patient comfort and informed consent is the cornerstone of the ethical practice of minimally invasive anesthesia.

This holistic perspective emphasizes the importance of viewing minimally invasive anesthesia not just as a collection of isolated techniques, but as a comprehensive approach focused on the patient's overall well-being. It involves a coordinated effort that begins with preoperative assessment and extends to postoperative care, guided by the principles of patient safety, ethical practice, and a commitment to optimal outcomes. In essence, it's about providing the best possible care in the least invasive manner.

1.2 Benefits of Minimally Invasive Approaches

Smaller incisions mean less trauma. This translates directly to less pain for the patient, a significantly improved experience from the initial procedure through recovery. Reduced tissue damage also minimizes the risk of complications, such as infection or excessive bleeding, contributing to a safer overall outcome. We're talking about a tangible improvement in the patient's quality of life, not just a theoretical one.

Faster recovery times are a major advantage. Patients undergoing minimally invasive procedures often experience a quicker return to their normal activities. This is due to the reduced trauma and the smaller surgical site that requires less healing. Reduced hospital stays and their associated costs are a welcome benefit for both patients and healthcare systems. Discharge planning becomes streamlined, leading to a quicker return to home and familiar surroundings for accelerated healing.

Minimally invasive techniques often lead to shorter hospital stays.

This decreases the risk of healthcare-associated infections, a serious concern in any surgical setting. Shorter hospital stays also mean reduced overall healthcare costs, both for the individual patient and the system as a whole. Consider the implications for patients' financial burdens, and the impact on healthcare resource allocation. The financial benefits are significant and should not be overlooked.

Reduced scarring is another considerable benefit. The smaller incisions characteristic of minimally invasive procedures result in smaller and less noticeable scars. This is particularly important for patients who are self-conscious about the appearance of surgical scars. It boosts patient confidence, and psychological well-being post-procedure. The aesthetic aspect should not be underestimated; it's a critical factor in patient satisfaction.

The overall improved patient experience, including less pain, faster recovery, and reduced scarring, contributes to increased patient satisfaction. Patients are more likely to be satisfied with the care they receive if their experience is positive and less traumatic. This satisfaction then translates to better adherence to post-operative instructions, leading to a higher success rate in treatment and improved long-term outcomes. A satisfied patient is a cooperative patient; this is essential for optimal recovery and treatment success.

Enhanced precision is a hallmark of minimally invasive surgery. Advanced imaging techniques and specialized instruments allow surgeons to perform the procedure with greater accuracy, reducing the risk of collateral damage to surrounding tissues and organs. This improved precision results in more effective treatment, and minimizes the potential for complications. A key element in successful minimally invasive procedures is the precise targeting of the surgical area.

Minimally invasive techniques often allow for earlier mobilization and a faster return to work. Reduced pain and faster recovery times make it easier for patients to resume normal activities more quickly. This has significant implications for patients' quality of life, especially for those who rely on their physical capabilities for work or other activities. The economic implications for the patient and society are noteworthy, enhancing productivity and overall economic output.

Improved cosmetic outcomes are a common consequence of these techniques. Besides reduced scarring, the smaller incisions often lead to a better overall cosmetic appearance. This is particularly important for procedures in visible areas. The improved aesthetic outcomes contribute to better patient self-esteem and body image after the procedure. Patient satisfaction directly correlates to psychological and emotional well-being.

Because of less tissue trauma, patients often experience less postoperative pain. This reduction in pain means patients require less pain medication, decreasing the risk of side effects related to analgesics. Less reliance on opioid medications is crucial, helping to mitigate the risk of addiction and other complications associated with prolonged opioid use. It's a significant factor in improving patient safety.

The reduction in complications, coupled with faster recovery, often translates into decreased overall healthcare costs. Shorter hospital stays, reduced need for pain medication, and lower risk of post-surgical issues all contribute to a more efficient and cost-effective approach to patient care. This is not just good for the patients but also for healthcare systems facing increasing budget constraints. It's a win-win for everyone involved.

2 Sedation Methods Overview

Conscious sedation, often involving a combination of anxiolytics and analgesics, allows patients to maintain their airway reflexes and respond to verbal commands. This approach is suitable for procedures with minimal discomfort, enabling patients to cooperate and participate actively, reducing anxiety and post-procedural distress. Careful monitoring of vital signs, including heart rate, blood pressure, and oxygen saturation, is crucial, as is the presence of trained personnel capable of managing potential complications. Midazolam, a benzodiazepine, is frequently used for its anxiolytic and amnestic properties, while opioids, like fentanyl, can provide analgesia. The skillful combination of these medications, tailored to the patient's individual needs and the procedure's demands, is paramount to a successful outcome. Maintaining patient safety throughout the process is of the utmost importance, including post-procedure observation for any adverse reactions.

Moderate sedation, also known as procedural sedation and analgesia, requires a more profound level of sedation than conscious sedation. Patients in this state are responsive to verbal commands but may not be fully oriented to time and place. While the airway remains protected, closer monitoring is essential, with the potential need for intervention to maintain respiratory function. Propofol, a commonly used intravenous anesthetic, provides rapid onset and short duration of action, making it ideal for brief procedures. However, its use requires experienced professionals due to its potential to depress respiration. Careful attention must be given to maintaining adequate oxygenation and ventilation; continuous pulse oximetry and capnography are crucial components of monitoring. The selection of medications and their dosages must be carefully considered, adapting to factors such as patient age, weight, and underlying medical conditions. Recovery from moderate sedation is generally swift, although continued monitoring is necessary until the patient has fully regained consciousness and motor control.

Deep sedation represents the most profound level of sedation, wherein patients are unresponsive to verbal commands and require assistance in maintaining their airway. This level of sedation demands significantly more intense monitoring and potential interventions. The risks of respiratory depression and hypotension increase substantially. Intravenous anesthetics, such as propofol and etomidate, are often used in conjunction with opioids and other medications to achieve the desired level of sedation. The airway management, possibly including endotracheal intubation, might be needed to ensure adequate oxygenation and ventilation. Continuous monitoring of vital signs, including heart rate, blood pressure, oxygen saturation, and end-tidal carbon dioxide, is mandatory. The patient's hemodynamic status must be constantly monitored, and interventions, such as fluid administration or vasopressors, might be necessary to counteract hypotension. A dedicated anesthesia team is imperative for managing deep sedation, and the selection of the patient for this level of sedation should be carefully considered based on procedural need and patient risk assessment. Detailed postoperative care, including close observation for complications, is crucial for a safe and complete recovery. Only trained and experienced medical professionals should perform this procedure. Even with careful planning and skilled management, complications can arise, emphasizing the need for prompt and appropriate interventions to ensure patient safety.

The selection of a particular sedation method hinges upon several interconnected factors. Firstly, the nature of the procedure itself plays a significant role; simple, short procedures might only necessitate conscious sedation, whereas extensive or more invasive procedures might necessitate moderate or even deep sedation. Secondly, the patient's overall health, pre-existing medical conditions, and any potential drug interactions must be carefully evaluated. Thirdly, the patient's preferences and anxieties need to be considered, taking into account their emotional state and readiness for the procedure. Lastly, the availability of resources and personnel within the healthcare setting will influence the feasible sedation options. A careful assessment of all these factors enables clinicians to make well-informed choices, ensuring that the selected sedation method maximizes patient comfort and safety whilst maintaining the success of the procedure. Remember, the primary goal remains a safe and effective procedure with minimal discomfort for the patient. Choosing an appropriate method requires a deep understanding of each technique's capabilities and limitations, alongside comprehensive patient assessment. Therefore, a collaborative approach between clinicians and patient is essential to achieve optimal outcomes.

2.1 Conscious Sedation Techniques

Conscious sedation allows patients to maintain a degree of responsiveness while experiencing reduced anxiety and discomfort. This is achieved through a careful balance of sedative and analgesic medications, tailored to the individual patient's needs and the specifics of the procedure. Careful monitoring is paramount, ensuring patient safety throughout the process.

The selection of sedative agents is crucial, with factors such as the patient's medical history, age, and the type of procedure heavily influencing the choice. Commonly used medications include benzodiazepines, such as midazolam, which provide anxiolysis and mild sedation, and opioids, like fentanyl, offering analgesia and further sedation. The administration route–intravenous, intramuscular, or intranasal–is also determined by individual circumstances and the overall clinical setting.

Understanding the pharmacodynamics and pharmacokinetics of the chosen sedative is essential for safe and effective conscious sedation. Benzodiazepines, for instance, act on GABA receptors in the brain, enhancing inhibitory neurotransmission and producing a calming effect. Opioids, conversely, bind to opioid receptors, reducing pain perception and potentially inducing drowsiness. Knowing the onset, duration, and potential side effects of each drug allows for precise titration and effective monitoring.

Proper monitoring techniques are non-negotiable. Continuous monitoring of vital signs, including heart rate, blood pressure, respiratory rate, and oxygen saturation, is critical. Pulse oximetry is routinely used to track oxygen levels, allowing for timely intervention if saturation drops. Capnography, while not always necessary, offers valuable information about ventilation and can detect respiratory depression early on. Regular neurological assessments, noting levels of responsiveness and orientation, are equally crucial to ensure the patient's safety and comfort throughout the procedure.

Careful attention to patient selection is a critical element of successful conscious sedation. Patients with certain medical conditions, such as severe respiratory disease or compromised cardiac function, might be poor candidates. A thorough pre-procedure assessment, including a comprehensive history and physical examination, is essential. This assessment will identify potential risks and allow for appropriate adjustments to the sedation plan. Any history of drug allergies must be carefully noted, and suitable alternative medications considered if necessary. Preoperative instructions to the patient and their caregiver are also vital, clearly outlining the procedure, potential side effects, and post-procedure care guidelines. Informed consent is paramount, ensuring that the patient understands the risks and benefits before proceeding.

Post-procedure care is equally important to the patient's well-being and safety. Patients need to be closely monitored until they are fully awake and alert, with clear guidelines on when they can be discharged from the facility. Post-sedation instructions should include recommendations on hydration, nutrition, and activity levels to support a safe and effective recovery. Patients should be advised to avoid driving or operating machinery for a specified period following sedation to ensure safety. A clear and concise follow-up plan, including contact information for any issues or concerns, needs to be clearly laid out for the patient and their support system. This ensures effective communication and promotes patient safety.

Beyond the immediate post-procedure period, long-term considerations are also important. Following up with patients, especially for procedures involving longer recovery times, helps assess the ongoing effects of the sedation and allows for the identification and management of any potential delayed complications. Regular follow-up allows the practitioner to obtain feedback on the effectiveness of the procedure and adjust their approach for future procedures. This is a crucial aspect of optimizing patient care and improving practice standards over time. Continuous learning and adherence to best practices, including staying up-to-date on the latest guidelines and protocols, remain paramount for healthcare professionals involved in conscious sedation. Such dedication to professional development ensures optimal patient safety and outcomes. The aim is not just effective sedation but also optimal patient experience and recovery.

Maintaining a meticulous record of each conscious sedation procedure is crucial for both legal and professional reasons. Thorough documentation of the patient's history, the medications used, monitoring data, any complications encountered, and the post-procedure recovery is essential. This complete and accurate documentation offers a valuable source of information for reviewing past cases, improving clinical practice, and ensuring compliance with regulatory standards. It also protects the clinician and the facility from potential liability by providing a detailed account of the care provided. Maintaining up-to-date and precise records demonstrates a dedication to both patient safety and professional responsibility.

2.2 Moderate Sedation Protocols

Moderate sedation allows patients to maintain their own airway and respond to verbal commands, a crucial difference from deeper sedation levels. This controlled state minimizes discomfort while ensuring the patient's safety. Achieving this balance requires meticulous attention to detail and a thorough understanding of the medications used and their potential effects. The key is careful titration of drugs, constant monitoring, and a rapid response to any adverse events.

Selecting the appropriate sedative depends greatly on the procedure's length and invasiveness, the patient's medical history, and their individual response to medications. Common choices include benzodiazepines, such as midazolam, known for their anxiolytic and amnestic properties, or opioids, such as fentanyl, effective in managing pain and providing additional sedation. However, the combined use of both classes presents a risk of respiratory depression, necessitating vigilant monitoring. Therefore, a clear understanding of drug interactions and potential synergistic effects is paramount. The initial dose should always be conservative, followed by incremental adjustments based on the patient's response.

Continuous monitoring is the cornerstone of safe moderate sedation. This includes close observation of vital signs—heart rate, blood pressure, respiratory rate, and oxygen saturation—using pulse oximetry and non-invasive blood pressure cuffs. Cardiac monitoring, although not always strictly required, provides additional reassurance, especially in patients with pre-existing cardiac conditions. Regular assessment of the patient's responsiveness—checking their ability to follow simple commands— is crucial to detect any signs of deepening sedation. Promptly adjusting medication dosage or providing supportive measures like supplemental oxygen is crucial in preventing complications. Establishing clear communication pathways between the sedation provider, the procedure operator, and the nursing staff is absolutely vital. Effective communication minimizes delays in responding to unexpected events, enhancing patient safety. A designated individual should be solely focused on monitoring the patient's status, allowing the other personnel to concentrate on their respective tasks. This collaborative approach ensures comprehensive care and facilitates a smooth procedural course, especially during longer or more complex interventions. Regular briefings on the patient's condition, including any significant changes, should occur to maintain everyone involved on the same page.

Recovery from moderate sedation should be carefully managed. Patients should be monitored until they have regained their full alertness and protective reflexes. This often involves observing them for several hours post-procedure, ensuring they can safely ambulate and that any residual effects of the sedatives have subsided. The provision of clear post-procedure instructions, including warnings about possible drowsiness and driving restrictions, is essential for patient safety and successful discharge. Before discharging the patient, it's important to assess whether there is a responsible adult who can accompany them home and provide ongoing supervision until they are fully recovered. Post-procedure complications, while rare with proper management, can include respiratory depression, hypotension, and nausea. Therefore, preparedness is key. The availability of resuscitation equipment and trained personnel capable of managing these emergencies is mandatory. Protocols should be established to clearly define the actions to be taken in the event of any complication. Regular drills and simulations should be conducted to ensure the team's proficiency in handling such situations. This proactive approach minimizes risks and optimizes patient safety, making for an excellent quality outcome. Remember, comprehensive training and regular procedural refinement are crucial for mastering moderate sedation.

The success of moderate sedation hinges on a combination of factors, encompassing skillful drug administration, careful monitoring, effective communication, and prompt response to complications. Adherence to established protocols, combined with vigilance and adaptability, allows clinicians to provide patients with a safe and comfortable procedural experience. Never underestimate the importance of ongoing education and a commitment to continuous improvement in your practice. Consistent attention to these aspects ensures both the patient's well-being and the maintenance of high-quality standards. Continuous learning about new advancements and strategies is crucial to maintain proficiency.

By thoroughly understanding and implementing these protocols, healthcare professionals can safely utilize moderate sedation to improve patient comfort and procedural outcomes. Remember, the primary objective is always the patient's safety and well-being, so diligent attention to these principles is not merely recommended but absolutely imperative. Always strive for excellence in your practice and continue your education, as even the most experienced professionals stand to benefit from refined knowledge and skills. Remember that patient care is a continuous learning process that requires ongoing commitment and improvement.

2.3 Deep Sedation Considerations

Deep sedation requires meticulous planning and execution. It's not a casual decision; careful consideration of the patient's medical history, including allergies, current medications, and any pre-existing conditions like heart or lung disease, is paramount. This comprehensive assessment helps predict potential complications and guide the selection of appropriate sedatives and monitoring strategies. A thorough understanding of the patient's overall health is crucial for ensuring their safety.

The choice of sedative agents is equally critical. Propofol, for instance, is a commonly used agent known for its rapid onset and short duration of action, making it suitable for short procedures. However, it can suppress respiration, necessitating close monitoring of vital signs. Other options, like etomidate or midazolam, may be preferred depending on the specific needs of the procedure and the patient's individual characteristics. Understanding the pharmacokinetic and pharmacodynamic profiles of these agents is essential for safe and effective administration.

Monitoring during deep sedation is not simply observing; it's actively safeguarding the patient's well-being. Continuous monitoring of vital signs, including heart rate, blood pressure, respiratory rate, and oxygen saturation, is mandatory. Pulse oximetry provides a continuous assessment of oxygen levels, while capnography offers real-time monitoring of carbon dioxide levels, reflecting respiratory function. Electrocardiography (ECG) continuously monitors the heart's electrical activity, aiding in the detection of any cardiac irregularities that may arise. These monitoring techniques are crucial for promptly identifying and addressing any adverse events.

Respiratory depression is a significant risk associated with deep sedation, demanding vigilant observation. The administration of supplemental oxygen is often necessary, and in cases of severe respiratory compromise, mechanical ventilation may be required. Having the necessary equipment readily available and a clear plan for managing respiratory depression is crucial to prevent serious complications. The team must be prepared to intervene quickly and decisively to restore adequate respiratory function.

Maintaining hemodynamic stability is equally important. Hypotension, a common side effect of some sedative agents, requires immediate attention. Fluid resuscitation, often with intravenous fluids, is typically the first line of defense. In more severe cases, vasopressor medications may be necessary to raise blood pressure and maintain adequate tissue perfusion. Careful titration of sedative agents and the use of appropriate supportive measures can mitigate this risk effectively.

Post-sedation care is just as important as the procedure itself. Patients require careful observation to ensure a smooth recovery. Maintaining an airway and monitoring vital signs are essential. The recovery phase may include measures to counteract the effects of sedation, such as administering fluids and closely monitoring their breathing until normal function returns. The time a patient remains under observation varies depending on the type of sedative and the nature of the procedure.

The management of potential complications should be proactively planned before the procedure. Anticipating potential problems, such as allergic reactions or unexpected changes in the patient's condition, allows for a more effective response and better patient outcomes. Having pre-established protocols for managing these situations can greatly improve patient safety. A clear understanding of the different kinds of complications related to each sedative agent helps in mitigating risks.

Deep sedation is a powerful tool, but it carries inherent risks. The use of deep sedation should always be justified by the clinical necessity. The benefits of the procedure must outweigh the inherent risks, and the procedure must be performed by a suitably qualified and experienced team. This approach ensures patient safety and optimal outcomes. The safety and well-being of the patient should always be the priority.

Choosing the right team is as essential as the right equipment. The administering physician and the supporting personnel must have the proper training and expertise in deep sedation, ensuring a safe and successful outcome for the patient. This is critical because any unforeseen issues can be easily managed. A well-coordinated team working together effectively contributes to the patient's safety.

Legal and ethical considerations are also crucial. Informed consent is paramount; patients must understand the procedure, its risks, and potential benefits before agreeing to deep sedation. Maintaining comprehensive documentation of the procedure, including the medications used, dosages, and the patient's response, is a vital aspect of responsible clinical practice, protecting both the patient and the medical team.

This includes recording any changes in the patient's condition or unexpected reactions during and after the sedation. This documentation can be used for future reference and potential analysis.
The benefits of deep sedation, when appropriately applied, significantly enhance patient comfort and facilitate the execution of necessary procedures. The successful utilization of deep sedation is dependent upon the conscientious application of the principles outlined above. By carefully considering patient selection, medication choice, monitoring techniques, and thorough post-procedure care, a safe and beneficial outcome can be ensured. Always remember the patient's well-being is the primary goal, shaping every decision in the process.

3 Local Anesthesia Techniques

Precise needle placement is paramount. A thorough understanding of regional anatomy, including nerve pathways and vascular structures, is crucial for successful nerve blocks. Consider using ultrasound guidance, especially for complex blocks, improving accuracy and minimizing the risk of complications like nerve injury or hematoma formation. Remember, patient positioning is also key; proper positioning facilitates accurate needle placement and patient comfort. Always aspirate before injecting to avoid intravascular injection.

Accurate and efficient infiltration anesthesia depends heavily on the spread of anesthetic solution. The injection technique significantly influences the extent of anesthesia achieved. Multiple small injections, rather than a single large injection, may provide more even distribution, especially in areas with dense tissue. The choice of anesthetic agent also plays a crucial role; some agents provide a longer duration of anesthesia, which is important for extended procedures. Always prioritize patient comfort; slow and gradual injection minimizes discomfort during the procedure.

Regional anesthesia offers broader pain control than infiltration techniques. Techniques such as brachial plexus blocks provide anesthesia to an entire limb. Thorough knowledge of relevant anatomy is essential for effective regional blocks, enabling precise targeting of nerve bundles. The choice between different regional anesthesia techniques, such as peripheral nerve blocks or epidural anesthesia, hinges on the specific surgical site and the patient's overall health. Remember to always consider potential complications; for instance, spinal headache is a possibility with epidural anesthesia. Post-procedural monitoring and follow-up are vital for early detection and management of complications.

Topical anesthesia, often used for superficial procedures, offers a simple and non-invasive approach. Eutectic mixture of local anesthetics (EMLA) cream is frequently used, applying a sufficient amount to the target area well in advance to allow for adequate penetration. The duration of action of topical anesthesia varies, influencing the preparation time needed before the procedure. It's vital to remember that the effectiveness of topical anesthesia can be affected by skin condition and the site of application, warranting an appropriate selection of anesthetic agent for optimal results. This method provides a convenient, minimal-discomfort option for certain procedures.

Combining different anesthesia techniques can provide enhanced pain control and patient comfort. For instance, combining a nerve block with infiltration anesthesia might offer comprehensive anesthesia for more extensive procedures. This combined approach offers flexibility, adjusting the type and dose of anesthetic agents based on the individual needs of the patient and the procedure's complexity. However, careful consideration of the interaction between different anesthetics is essential to prevent adverse reactions. Always prioritize patient safety when utilizing a combined approach, monitoring for signs of toxicity or other complications.

Accurate documentation is vital, regardless of the chosen anesthesia method. This includes the type and amount of anesthetic agent used, the injection sites, any complications encountered, and the patient's response to the anesthesia. Clear and complete documentation protects both the patient and the healthcare provider, aiding in quality improvement initiatives and preventing potential legal issues. Accurate and thorough records ensure continuity of care, enabling efficient communication between medical professionals involved in the patient's care. This commitment to detailed records underlines a commitment to responsible practice.

3.1 Nerve Blocks: Principles & Practice

Nerve blocks offer a powerful tool in minimally invasive anesthesia, providing excellent analgesia with reduced systemic effects compared to general anesthesia. Understanding the underlying principles–specifically, the precise location and distribution of nerves–is paramount for successful and safe administration. Accurate anatomical knowledge, coupled with a meticulous approach, directly impacts the effectiveness of the block and minimizes the risk of complications. This includes a comprehensive understanding of relevant neuroanatomy and the targeted nerves' innervation patterns. For example, a thorough understanding of the brachial plexus is essential for performing successful upper limb blocks.

Effective nerve blocks depend heavily on the proper selection of local anesthetic agents and the precise injection technique. The choice of agent should consider factors such as the duration of the procedure, the patient's medical history (including allergies and potential contraindications), and the specific nerves being targeted. Furthermore, the concentration of the anesthetic is crucial; higher concentrations may provide faster onset but can also increase the risk of systemic toxicity. The injection technique itself–whether ultrasound-guided or landmark-based–significantly influences the success rate. Ultrasound guidance, in particular, offers real-time visualization, significantly increasing accuracy and reducing the chance of inadvertent needle placement. Careful attention to asepsis throughout the procedure remains essential for preventing infection.

Beyond the immediate technique, patient preparation plays a crucial role in successful nerve blocks. This involves a detailed medical history, identifying any pre-existing conditions which might influence anesthetic choices or the procedure's outcome. This assessment includes identifying any potential contraindications to regional anesthesia. A thorough discussion about the procedure, including potential benefits, risks, and alternatives, is imperative to secure informed consent and alleviate patient anxiety. Preoperative assessments may also encompass blood tests to ascertain the patient's suitability for regional anesthetic techniques and identify potential risks, allowing adjustments to the procedure if needed. Premedication, though not always required, can play a crucial role in managing patient anxiety.

Post-procedure care is equally important as the procedure itself. Monitoring the patient closely for any signs of complications–such as local anesthetic systemic toxicity, hematoma formation, nerve injury, or infection–is crucial. Pain management is paramount; a tailored analgesic plan should address potential post-block pain, utilizing appropriate medications and monitoring their efficacy. Patient education is vital, as instructing the patient on potential post-block sensations and symptoms, including warning signs of complications, empowers them to actively participate in their own recovery. Thorough documentation of the procedure, including the type and amount of anesthetic used, the injection sites, and any complications encountered, is essential for maintaining accurate records and facilitates better patient management.

Several factors can influence the effectiveness of a nerve block. The patient's body habitus–including obesity or specific anatomical variations–can significantly affect needle placement accuracy. Certain medical conditions, such as peripheral neuropathy, can also alter the response to local anesthetic agents. Additionally, variations in individual patient responses to medications should always be considered. Careful attention to detail in all phases of the procedure remains paramount. Incorporating advanced techniques like ultrasound guidance consistently improves the accuracy of nerve localization and minimizes the incidence of complications, improving patient outcomes and leading to better procedural success rates. This technological innovation has revolutionized the practice of nerve blocks, significantly enhancing their safety and efficacy.

The successful application of nerve blocks requires ongoing learning and refinement of technique. Continuous professional development, including participation in workshops and staying updated with the latest research and best practices, is crucial. Learning from experienced practitioners provides invaluable insights into practical skills and troubleshooting techniques. Regular self-assessment and the review of individual cases are invaluable means of continually improving performance and identifying areas for further improvement. Ultimately, mastery of nerve block techniques necessitates ongoing dedication, commitment to continuous learning and improvement, and a consistent focus on patient safety. This careful approach ensures that we provide patients with the safest and most effective pain management solutions.

3.2 Infiltration Anesthesia Methods

Infiltration anesthesia involves injecting a local anesthetic solution directly into the tissues surrounding the surgical site. This technique is straightforward, relatively quick, and often provides adequate analgesia for minor procedures. It's a cornerstone of many minimally invasive techniques, offering a valuable tool for managing patient discomfort.

The choice of anesthetic agent depends greatly on the procedure and the patient's individual needs. Lidocaine, bupivacaine, and ropivacaine are frequently used, each possessing unique properties concerning duration of action and potential side effects. Careful consideration of these factors is essential for optimal patient care. Understanding the pharmacokinetic and pharmacodynamic profiles of these agents is crucial for safe and effective administration.

Proper technique is paramount. The injection should be slow and deliberate to minimize discomfort and potential complications, such as hematoma formation or inadvertent intravascular injection. Using a fine-gauge needle further reduces patient discomfort and risk. Aspiration before injection is a critical step to ensure the needle isn't within a blood vessel. Failure to do so can lead to systemic toxicity, a serious adverse event. Moreover, spreading the anesthetic solution across the target area, rather than injecting it in a single location, helps ensure wider coverage and pain relief.

Specific anatomical considerations are essential for effective infiltration. Knowing the location of major nerves and blood vessels is paramount to avoid complications. Careful palpation and visualization of the surgical site are crucial steps in the process. Detailed anatomical knowledge, honed through experience and continuing education, allows practitioners to perform infiltrations safely and effectively, minimizing the risk of complications.

Preoperative patient assessment is equally important. A complete review of the patient's medical history, including allergies and potential drug interactions, is essential. Understanding the patient's expectations and anxieties can help manage their pain experience, contributing to a positive outcome. Open communication with the patient, answering any questions or concerns, establishes trust and allows for a more collaborative approach to the procedure.

Post-procedure monitoring is an integral part of safe infiltration anesthesia. Observing the patient for signs of local anesthetic toxicity, such as lightheadedness, dizziness, or tingling, is crucial. Monitoring vital signs, such as heart rate and blood pressure, allows for early detection and management of any adverse events. Prompt intervention in case of complications significantly reduces the risk of severe outcomes. Furthermore, providing the patient with clear post-procedure instructions, including advice on managing potential discomfort and when to seek medical attention, is vital for a successful outcome.

While infiltration anesthesia is generally safe, complications can occur. These can range from relatively minor events, such as bruising or localized swelling, to more serious ones, like nerve injury or systemic toxicity. Understanding these potential complications and having a plan to manage them is critical. Moreover, being prepared for allergic reactions is also crucial; having appropriate medications available and knowing how to manage anaphylaxis can be lifesaving.

The efficacy of infiltration anesthesia can vary depending on the procedure's complexity and the patient's individual factors. For example, highly innervated tissues may require higher concentrations of anesthetic or the addition of other adjunctive techniques like nerve blocks or topical anesthetics. Understanding these limitations helps in choosing the most appropriate anesthetic strategy.

Continual professional development is crucial in mastering infiltration anesthesia techniques. Staying updated on the latest research, best practices, and advancements in anesthetic agents allows for the delivery of the safest and most effective care. Regular review of rele-

vant literature and participation in continuing education courses are essential for maintaining competence and improving patient outcomes. Regular self-assessment and reflection on the efficacy and safety of the procedures performed are vital for continued professional growth.
In summary, infiltration anesthesia remains a crucial technique in minimally invasive procedures, offering a simple yet effective method for managing pain. However, achieving optimal results requires a thorough understanding of the relevant anatomy, appropriate anesthetic agent selection, meticulous injection techniques, comprehensive patient assessment, and proactive post-procedure monitoring. Continual professional development and the adoption of safe practices are vital to minimizing risks and maximizing patient comfort and safety.

3.3 Regional Anesthesia Techniques

Regional anesthesia involves injecting local anesthetic near a nerve or group of nerves, effectively numbing a specific body region. This targeted approach minimizes systemic exposure to the anesthetic, leading to fewer side effects compared to general anesthesia. The technique's precision allows for surgical procedures or other interventions with significantly reduced discomfort and faster recovery times for the patient.
Unlike general anesthesia, which affects the entire body, regional anesthesia allows patients to remain conscious or only mildly sedated. This consciousness can be advantageous, allowing for easier communication and quicker assessment of the patient's well-being during the procedure. Moreover, the avoidance of general anesthesia's potential complications, such as respiratory depression and nausea, makes regional anesthesia a safer and often preferred option, especially for specific patient populations.

Preparation for regional anesthesia begins with a comprehensive assessment of the patient. This involves a thorough review of medical history, including any allergies, current medications, and pre-existing conditions that might influence the anesthetic's effect or increase the risk of complications. A detailed explanation of the procedure, its benefits, risks, and alternatives, is crucial to obtain informed consent. This underscores the ethical responsibility of the practitioner and the importance of patient autonomy.

Several regional anesthesia techniques exist, each tailored to a specific anatomical area. For example, brachial plexus blocks numb the arm, while femoral nerve blocks affect the leg. Epidural anesthesia, administered in the epidural space of the spine, provides broader regional anesthesia, frequently used for labor pain management and lower limb surgery. The choice of technique depends on several factors, including the procedure's location, the patient's overall health, and the anesthesiologist's expertise.

Mastering the techniques requires meticulous attention to detail. Accurate landmark identification is essential to ensure the anesthetic reaches the target nerves without affecting adjacent structures. Ultrasound guidance is increasingly used to visualize nerves and confirm accurate needle placement, minimizing the risk of accidental injury. Continuous monitoring of the patient's vital signs, including heart rate, blood pressure, and oxygen saturation, is essential throughout the procedure and recovery period.

Post-procedure care involves close monitoring for any signs of complications, such as bleeding, infection, or nerve damage. Pain management after regional anesthesia is often less intense than after general anesthesia, potentially decreasing the need for strong opioids. Patient education about expected sensations, potential side effects, and appropriate post-procedural care is crucial to ensure a smooth recovery and prevent unnecessary complications. Careful attention must be given to monitoring for potential signs of nerve injury, and providing appropriate post-operative analgesia.

The successful application of regional anesthesia relies heavily on a strong understanding of anatomy, pharmacology, and patient physiology. It demands meticulous attention to detail in all stages, from pre-procedure assessment and preparation to the injection itself, and subsequent patient monitoring. Regular review of procedural protocols and continuous learning is imperative to enhance patient safety and optimize outcomes. The use of appropriate nerve stimulators and aspiration before injection further increases safety.

Furthermore, ongoing research continues to refine regional anesthesia techniques, exploring new anesthetic agents, improving injection methods, and developing advanced monitoring tools. This ongoing pursuit of improvement underscores the commitment to patient safety and the constant drive towards better patient outcomes, minimizing pain and discomfort throughout the procedural and post-procedural phases. It is crucial for practitioners to stay abreast of these advancements to provide optimal care. Continued learning and adherence to safety protocols are crucial aspects of practicing regional anesthesia effectively and safely.

To conclude, regional anesthesia represents a significant advancement in minimally invasive pain management. Its benefits extend beyond simple pain relief to encompass enhanced patient safety, reduced side effects, and quicker recovery times. However, responsible and effective utilization requires extensive knowledge, meticulous technique, and commitment to ongoing professional development. The potential complications of regional anesthesia highlight the need for meticulous attention to detail and a comprehensive understanding of the relevant anatomy and physiology. This is crucial in ensuring the safety and well-being of patients undergoing procedures employing regional anesthesia.

3.4 Topical Anesthesia Applications

Topical anesthesia provides a valuable, often overlooked, tool in the minimally invasive anesthesia arsenal. Its simplicity belies its effectiveness, particularly in superficial procedures. Application is straightforward, requiring minimal equipment and training, making it ideal for various settings, from the clinic to the operating room.

The mechanism of action hinges on the disruption of nerve impulse transmission within the skin and mucous membranes. This is achieved by blocking sodium channels, thereby preventing the propagation of pain signals to the central nervous system. The choice of anesthetic agent depends largely on the specific procedure and patient factors. Lidocaine and tetracaine are common choices, often combined with epinephrine for vasoconstriction, prolonging the anesthetic effect and reducing bleeding. Benzocaine, a less potent but readily available option, finds use in certain applications.

Careful application technique is crucial for optimal results. The area to be anesthetized should be cleaned thoroughly before application. Excess hair should be removed, promoting better contact with the skin. The anesthetic cream or gel should be applied liberally and evenly, covering the entire target area, extending slightly beyond the surgical field. A thin layer of occlusive dressing can enhance penetration and prolong the anesthetic effect. The required contact time varies with the agent and concentration, ranging from 15 minutes to an hour.

Monitoring the patient's response is essential. While generally considered safe, topical anesthetics can cause adverse reactions. These can range from mild, such as local skin irritation and burning, to more severe reactions, including systemic toxicity. Careful observation for signs of allergic reactions, such as rash, itching, or swelling, is paramount. Any signs of systemic toxicity, such as dizziness, lightheadedness, or cardiovascular changes, should be treated immediately. Rapid pulse, arrhythmia or respiratory changes warrant immediate attention.

Patient education plays a vital role. Before the procedure, patients should be informed about the process, potential benefits, and associated risks. They should be specifically instructed on what to expect during the application, including any potential sensations, such as minor stinging or burning. Post-procedure, patients need to understand the importance of maintaining the integrity of the application site to prevent infection and promote healing. Clear instructions on wound care should be provided, and patients should be educated on recognizing potential complications and when to seek medical attention.

Combining topical anesthesia with other minimally invasive techniques can result in synergistic effects. For example, combining topical anesthesia with a nerve block can provide more extensive pain relief for certain procedures. This combined approach can be particularly useful in cases requiring both superficial and deeper anesthesia. Similarly, topical anesthesia can complement conscious sedation by providing supplemental local analgesia, reducing the overall requirement for systemic sedatives and minimizing their associated risks.

The selection of appropriate topical anesthetic must be guided by patient-specific factors. Pre-existing conditions, such as allergies or cardiovascular disease, may influence the choice of agent and concentration. The patient's age and overall health should also be taken into consideration. Detailed assessment and evaluation of the patient's suitability for topical anesthesia are therefore crucial.

Furthermore, the efficacy of topical anesthesia can be affected by various factors. Skin thickness, presence of inflammation or infection, and the type of procedure itself all play a role. In areas with thicker skin, such as the soles of the feet, higher concentrations or longer contact times may be necessary. Similarly, the presence of inflammation can reduce the effectiveness of topical anesthetics. An accurate assessment of these factors allows for adjustments to the anesthetic regimen, optimizing efficacy and minimizing side effects.

The widespread availability and ease of application make topical anesthesia a versatile tool. Its use extends across numerous specialties. Dermatology, ophthalmology, and dentistry routinely employ topical anesthetics for procedures requiring superficial analgesia. Beyond specific medical procedures, topical anesthetics find application in managing various conditions. Pain relief for minor burns, skin abrasions and certain types of chronic pain syndromes have all witnessed the benefit of topical application. This makes topical anesthesia a valuable resource for pain management in a variety of healthcare contexts.

The appropriate use of topical anesthesia demonstrates a commitment to patient-centered care. Minimizing discomfort and anxiety are paramount to positive patient outcomes. A careful approach, involving proper patient selection, informed consent, and meticulous application technique, ensures safe and effective pain management. Continuous monitoring and prompt management of any complications contribute to the overall success of the procedure and patient satisfaction.

3.5 Combined Anesthesia Approaches

Combining local anesthetic techniques with sedation offers a powerful strategy for managing pain and anxiety during minimally invasive procedures. This approach allows for a tailored anesthetic plan, optimizing patient comfort and minimizing the risks associated with either technique alone. For instance, a patient undergoing a minor surgical procedure might benefit from a local anesthetic nerve block combined with conscious sedation. The nerve block provides targeted pain relief, while the sedation helps reduce anxiety and promotes relaxation. This synergistic effect can significantly enhance the patient experience.

The selection of specific anesthetic agents depends heavily on the patient's individual needs and the nature of the procedure. Careful consideration of the patient's medical history, including allergies and drug interactions, is paramount. Preoperative assessment is crucial in identifying any potential contraindications or risks. This holistic approach ensures that the chosen combination is both effective and safe for the individual patient. Remember, thorough documentation of the anesthetic plan and its rationale is essential for maintaining clear communication and enabling future reference.

For example, consider a patient requiring a superficial wound repair. A combination of topical anesthesia with a mild sedative could suffice. The topical anesthetic numbs the skin surface, minimizing needle discomfort associated with local infiltration. Adding a sedative further reduces patient anxiety, leading to a more comfortable and cooperative experience throughout the procedure. This approach reduces the overall medication needed and allows for quicker patient recovery.

However, more complex procedures, like an arthroscopy, often demand a more comprehensive strategy. In such cases, a regional nerve block may be combined with moderate sedation. The nerve block provides extensive pain relief within the affected area, ensuring minimal discomfort during the procedure. Moderate sedation enhances relaxation and reduces procedural anxiety. Careful titration of sedation is crucial; it must alleviate anxiety without compromising the patient's airway or ability to respond to commands. Continuous monitoring of vital signs is necessary to detect any adverse effects and to ensure the

patient's safety throughout.
The potential benefits of combining local anesthetic techniques with sedation are numerous. Patients often experience reduced pain and discomfort, leading to improved satisfaction with the overall experience. Furthermore, the quicker recovery associated with minimally invasive anesthesia usually translates to shorter hospital stays and a faster return to normal activities. The reduced need for general anesthesia can significantly decrease the risk of complications such as nausea, vomiting, and post-operative cognitive dysfunction. Such outcomes, combined with higher patient satisfaction, are of significant value to both patients and healthcare professionals.
However, this approach isn't without potential challenges. Careful consideration of drug interactions is vital. Some sedatives, for instance, can potentiate the effects of local anesthetics, increasing the risk of systemic toxicity. Monitoring for signs of over-sedation, such as respiratory depression or hypotension, is absolutely crucial. The expertise of the anesthesiologist is essential in mitigating these risks, ensuring safe and effective patient management.
Accurate assessment of the patient's medical history and current condition precedes any combined anesthesia approach. This careful evaluation, coupled with an in-depth understanding of the procedure's specific needs, enables the creation of a personalized plan that balances efficacy with safety. The communication with the patient is also critical. Patients need to thoroughly understand the procedures, benefits, risks, and potential complications associated with each combined approach. This ensures informed consent and contributes to a positive overall experience. Remember, tailoring the anesthetic technique to the patient, not just the procedure, is crucial for success.
Finally, understanding the limitations of each technique is paramount. While combined approaches significantly enhance patient comfort,

they may not eliminate pain or anxiety entirely. It's imperative that physicians anticipate potential limitations and have backup plans in place to manage unexpected complications. The ability to swiftly adapt to changing circumstances is crucial in ensuring optimal patient safety and satisfaction throughout the entire procedure. Regular review and refinement of protocols based on the evolving landscape of minimally invasive anesthesia will lead to continued improvement in patient care. The field is constantly developing, and staying abreast of advancements is critical for professionals in this field.

4 Monitoring During Procedures

Continuous monitoring is paramount during minimally invasive procedures. It's not just about checking vital signs; it's about actively observing and interpreting the patient's response to the procedure and the administered medications. Think of it as a constant dialogue between the patient's body and your vigilance. Any deviation, however subtle, could indicate a developing complication that requires immediate attention. This proactive approach is the cornerstone of safe and effective minimally invasive anesthesia.

A comprehensive monitoring plan should include several key elements. First, continuous pulse oximetry is essential to track oxygen saturation levels. This simple yet critical tool provides real-time feedback on the patient's oxygenation status, alerting you to potential hypoxemia before it becomes clinically significant. Simultaneously, continuous monitoring of heart rate and rhythm is equally important, revealing any arrhythmias or bradycardia that might arise from the procedure or medication effects. Changes in heart rate can often precede more serious events, providing an early warning system. Blood pressure monitoring, ideally continuous, is also vital, as it provides insights into the patient's cardiovascular response to the procedure and the anesthetic agents used. Significant fluctuations in blood pressure necessitate immediate assessment and appropriate intervention.

Respiratory rate and pattern are also valuable indicators. Observing the depth and regularity of respiration helps detect early signs of respiratory depression, a potential complication of sedation. Any noticeable changes—shallow breathing, apnea, or irregular patterns—require prompt attention. Changes are sometimes subtle, requiring a keen eye and experienced observation, not just relying on numerical values. Beyond these key vital signs, consider supplementary monitoring depending on the specific procedure and patient characteristics. For instance, capnography, measuring the concentration of carbon dioxide in exhaled breath, can provide valuable insights into ventilation adequacy. Electrocardiogram (ECG) monitoring may be indicated in certain high-risk patients to detect potential cardiac complications.

The type of monitoring equipment used should reflect best practice guidelines and the individual needs of your patient. While sophisticated technologies can provide a wealth of information, the interpretation and application of this data is equally essential. Accurate interpretation requires experience, understanding, and quick reflexes to translate those data into real-time decision-making. Never rely solely on monitors; your clinical judgment remains the most critical tool in managing your patient's wellbeing. Observe the patient closely; observe subtle nuances such as skin color, sweating, or changes in behavior. These might indicate hypoxia, pain, or anxiety even before changes in vital signs appear.

Furthermore, consistent documentation of monitoring data is non-negotiable. Careful and precise record-keeping is critical for patient safety, legal protection, and continuous improvement. Accurate documentation allows for effective communication among healthcare professionals involved in the procedure. It also facilitates ongoing quality assurance reviews, offering opportunities to learn from previous experiences and refine your practice. Your records become a narrative of the procedural course, essential for future reference and analysis. Remember, every detail matters; every observation, every adjustment, every reaction, needs to be precisely recorded in the patient's chart, creating a complete picture of what occurred throughout the procedure. Consistent, accurate documentation helps paint a complete clinical picture that enhances patient safety and professional accountability. This should be seen as a cornerstone of your practice. The accuracy of your records significantly impacts patient safety, risk management, and regulatory compliance.

In conclusion, effective monitoring during minimally invasive procedures is a multi-faceted process that goes beyond simply checking vital signs. It requires a combination of technical proficiency, experienced clinical judgment, and a meticulous approach to record-keeping. By integrating these elements into your practice, you can proactively identify and manage potential complications, ensuring patient safety and optimal outcomes. The ultimate aim is to transform what might be a potentially painful or stressful experience into a safe and comfortable procedural pathway for the patient. Prioritizing vigilant, meticulous monitoring allows you to anticipate challenges and quickly adjust your approach, safeguarding both the patient and your professional practice.

4.1 Vital Sign Monitoring

Continuous monitoring is paramount during minimally invasive procedures. It allows for early detection of subtle changes, enabling timely intervention and preventing serious complications. This proactive approach significantly improves patient safety and outcomes. We must remember that even seemingly minor variations can indicate significant underlying issues. A vigilant approach is crucial.

Effective monitoring requires a systematic approach, encompassing both technological and observational elements. Reliable equipment is essential, but it's the clinician's keen observation and intuitive interpretation of data that ultimately guides decision-making. This combination is what ensures the best patient care. Never underestimate the power of carefully assessing a patient's overall condition.

Key vital signs to closely track include heart rate, blood pressure, respiratory rate, and oxygen saturation (SpO2). These parameters offer a comprehensive overview of the cardiovascular and respiratory systems. Consistent monitoring, noting trends and deviations from baseline values, is more valuable than isolated readings. Consider the patient's baseline health too; someone with pre-existing conditions may exhibit different "normal" ranges.

Variations in heart rate can indicate a wide array of issues, from hypovolemia to pain or anxiety. A sudden drop or increase should trigger immediate investigation and appropriate management, such as administering fluids or adjusting the anesthetic regimen. Remember that context is crucial; an increase in heart rate following a surgical incision could be normal for that patient.

Blood pressure monitoring is crucial, particularly in identifying potential hypotension or hypertension. These fluctuations can be influenced by various factors including the anesthetic agents used, fluid balance, and the surgical stress response. Maintaining a stable blood pressure is essential for adequate tissue perfusion and organ function. Close attention to any drops warrants immediate investigation, often involving increasing fluid administration.

Respiratory rate monitoring is equally vital, reflecting the patient's adequacy of ventilation and oxygenation. Changes in respiratory rate often precede more serious respiratory events. Any slowing or speeding up may necessitate careful observation, perhaps leading to adjustments in oxygen support or ventilatory support. Always consider the patient's pre-existing conditions and other medications when assessing.

Oxygen saturation (SpO2) provides a direct measure of arterial oxygenation. Maintaining adequate SpO2 is critical for preventing hypoxemia, a serious complication that can have significant consequences. Regular SpO2 monitoring ensures prompt identification and correction of any hypoxemic episodes, perhaps requiring supplemental oxygen. A persistent drop in SpO2 even with supplemental oxygen should raise immediate concern.

Beyond these fundamental vital signs, continuous electrocardiogram (ECG) monitoring is commonly recommended. This non-invasive technique provides real-time assessment of cardiac rhythm and electrical activity. ECG monitoring allows for early detection of arrhythmias and other cardiac issues, thus potentially preventing serious cardiac events. The importance of ECG interpretation skills for the procedural team cannot be overstated.

In addition to technological monitoring, your observation skills are essential. Pay close attention to the patient's level of consciousness, skin color, and any signs of distress, such as grimacing, restlessness or excessive sweating. These subtle cues can provide valuable insights that may not be immediately apparent from numerical data alone. Your eyes and intuition are as valuable as any instrument.

Finally, remember accurate documentation is essential. Maintain detailed records of all vital sign measurements, alongside any interventions taken, and any patient responses. This meticulous record-keeping enables careful analysis of patient progress and aids in identifying trends and patterns. This allows for improved care and is also important in risk management and medico-legal contexts. Thorough record keeping reflects professionalism and supports excellent patient care.

4.2 Oxygen Saturation Monitoring

Continuous monitoring of oxygen saturation (SpO2) is paramount during any minimally invasive procedure, regardless of the sedation level. A decline in SpO2, even a seemingly minor dip, can signal serious underlying issues requiring immediate attention. This is crucial because early intervention can prevent significant complications and ensure patient safety. Remember, prompt action is vital; delays can have severe repercussions.

Accurate SpO2 measurement relies on appropriate probe placement. The pulse oximeter probe should be securely attached to a fingertip, toe, or earlobe, ensuring good contact with the skin to obtain a reliable signal. Avoid applying the probe to areas with poor circulation or edema, as this could lead to inaccurate readings. Proper positioning minimizes interference and ensures accurate reflection of arterial oxygenation.

Interpretation of SpO2 readings needs to be done in context. While a reading below 95% generally indicates hypoxemia, other factors such as patient-specific conditions or the procedure itself should be considered. For example, a patient with chronic lung disease might have a baseline SpO2 slightly below 95%, therefore, any significant drop from their baseline would be concerning. Therefore, contextual understanding is vital in this practice.

Beyond the numerical value, observe the SpO2 waveform displayed on the monitor. A flat or erratic waveform could point to problems with probe placement or signal quality, even if the numerical reading appears acceptable. It is crucial to maintain continuous observation of these values and their quality. Any anomalies should prompt immediate attention. This involves checking probe placement, the quality of the signal, and exploring other potential causes.

Maintaining the integrity of the pulse oximeter equipment is also essential. Regular calibration and maintenance of the equipment are necessary to guarantee accurate and reliable readings. Familiarize yourself with the specifics of your equipment's maintenance schedule. Malfunctioning equipment can lead to inaccurate readings, potentially delaying the detection of critical complications.

SpO2 monitoring is only one aspect of overall patient surveillance during minimally invasive procedures. It should always be used in conjunction with other vital signs monitoring, such as heart rate, blood pressure, and respiratory rate, for a comprehensive picture of the patient's physiological state. Combining these parameters provides a more complete understanding of the patient's well-being.

Remember, SpO2 monitoring is not just about the number; it's about understanding the context, recognizing abnormalities in the waveform, and integrating this information with other clinical observations. This holistic approach is essential for the safe and successful completion of any minimally invasive procedure. Continuous vigilance is vital for optimal patient outcomes.

Effective communication is equally important. During a procedure, clear and concise communication between the anesthesia provider and the surgical team regarding SpO2 readings and any observed changes is essential. It's a collaborative effort. A proactive and consistent approach to communication will minimize any delay in intervention, enhancing patient safety.

Should SpO2 values consistently fall below the acceptable range despite appropriate probe placement and equipment function, consider potential causes such as hypoventilation, airway obstruction, or pulmonary embolism. If these issues are suspected, timely and appropriate interventions, such as supplemental oxygen, airway management techniques, or further diagnostic evaluation, may be necessary.

Documentation is a crucial final step. Meticulously record all SpO2 readings, any observed waveform irregularities, and any interventions undertaken in response to changes in SpO2 levels. This comprehensive record forms a valuable part of the patient's medical record, ensuring a complete account of the procedure and its associated monitoring parameters. Accuracy and completeness are key here to preserve patient safety and meet professional standards. Clear, concise, and accurate recording is vital.

5 Managing Complications

Hypotension, a common complication during minimally invasive procedures, necessitates prompt recognition and management. A sudden drop in blood pressure can be indicative of various underlying issues, including fluid loss, anesthetic effects, or allergic reactions. Careful monitoring of blood pressure, heart rate, and urine output is crucial. Initial management involves administering intravenous fluids, often crystalloids like normal saline, to expand the intravascular volume. If fluid resuscitation proves insufficient, vasopressors like epinephrine or norepinephrine may be needed, always titrated carefully to achieve the desired effect while avoiding excessive vasoconstriction. The underlying cause of the hypotension should be investigated concurrently.

Respiratory depression, characterized by decreased respiratory rate and depth, poses a serious risk during sedation and anesthesia. Early detection is paramount, relying heavily on vigilant monitoring of respiratory rate, oxygen saturation, and end-tidal carbon dioxide levels. If respiratory depression occurs, supplemental oxygen should be administered immediately, often via a face mask. If this is inadequate, positive pressure ventilation may be necessary, potentially through bag-valve mask ventilation or mechanical ventilation, depending on the severity of the situation and the available resources. Reversal agents, such as naloxone for opioid-induced respiratory depression, may be utilized if appropriate, always carefully considering the potential side effects and interactions with other medications. Maintaining airway patency is vital throughout the process.

Allergic reactions, ranging from mild skin rashes to life-threatening anaphylaxis, represent a significant challenge in procedural settings. Prompt recognition is critical; symptoms can manifest as urticaria, angioedema, bronchospasm, or hypotension. Immediate management involves discontinuing the offending agent, if possible. Oxygen administration is essential, and epinephrine is the cornerstone of treatment for anaphylaxis. This should be administered intravenously, with the dose tailored to the severity of the reaction according to established guidelines. Supportive care, including intravenous fluids and antihistamines, may be required to manage symptoms and prevent further complications. Close monitoring is crucial, and transferring the patient to a higher level of care may be necessary in severe cases.

Recognizing and addressing these complications requires a multifaceted approach. Proactive measures, such as a thorough pre-procedure assessment, accurate medication administration, and diligent monitoring, significantly reduce the likelihood of their occurrence. However, even with meticulous preparation, complications can arise. Rapid response teams and readily available emergency medications and equipment are essential components of a safe practice environment. A well-defined emergency protocol, practiced regularly and adhered to meticulously, ensures swift and effective intervention, thereby minimizing the potential for adverse outcomes. Furthermore, post-procedure monitoring and follow-up are equally vital aspects of managing complications and ensuring patient well-being. Continuous learning and staying abreast of the latest advances in anesthesia and sedation practices contribute to enhancing patient safety and improving outcomes.

Each complication demands immediate attention and a tailored approach. The severity of the complication will influence the speed and intensity of interventions. This involves accurate assessment, judicious selection of treatment modalities, and close monitoring to assess the effectiveness of interventions and to adjust accordingly. The focus must always remain on optimizing patient safety while mitigating potential risks. Effective communication amongst the medical team is also paramount in ensuring a coordinated and efficient response to any complications that might arise during minimally invasive procedures. Regular review of protocols and participation in relevant continuing medical education activities are critical for maintaining proficiency in managing potential complications and providing optimal patient care. The goal is always to ensure the procedure is as painless and safe as possible for the patient.

5.1 Hypotension Management

Hypotension, a decrease in blood pressure, is a potentially serious complication during minimally invasive procedures. Prompt recognition and effective management are crucial for patient safety. Failure to address hypotension can lead to inadequate tissue perfusion, organ damage, and even cardiac arrest. Therefore, understanding the causes, recognizing the symptoms, and implementing appropriate treatment strategies are paramount.

Several factors can contribute to intraoperative hypotension. These include the effects of anesthetic agents themselves, such as vasodilators or medications that depress cardiac function. Fluid shifts, stemming from changes in positioning or the procedure itself, can also significantly decrease blood volume, resulting in lower blood pressure. Additionally, anxiety and pain, even if minimized through the procedure's nature, can trigger the body's stress response, potentially leading to peripheral vasodilation and a subsequent drop in blood pressure. Pre-existing conditions like hypovolemia, cardiac dysfunction, or dehydration also increase a patient's risk.

Identifying hypotension involves constant monitoring of vital signs. Blood pressure, heart rate, and oxygen saturation are all crucial indicators. A sudden or gradual decrease in systolic blood pressure below the patient's baseline is the primary warning sign. Clinical signs, such as pallor, sweating, dizziness, and altered mental status, often accompany a significant drop in blood pressure and should prompt immediate intervention. These symptoms can manifest subtly, however, underscoring the importance of continuous and careful observation.

Management begins with identifying and addressing the underlying cause. The initial steps often involve optimizing fluid balance. Infusing intravenous fluids, such as crystalloids or colloids, can rapidly expand intravascular volume and restore blood pressure to safer levels. However, administering fluids must be done cautiously, considering the patient's overall condition and avoiding fluid overload. The rate of infusion is adjusted based on the patient's response to treatment, closely monitoring blood pressure and other vital signs.

If fluid resuscitation proves insufficient, vasopressor medications may be necessary. These drugs stimulate the sympathetic nervous system, increasing peripheral vascular resistance and raising blood pressure. The choice of vasopressor, such as ephedrine or phenylephrine, depends on the specific circumstances and the patient's response. Close monitoring of blood pressure, heart rate, and rhythm is essential during vasopressor administration to avoid excessive increases and potential complications. Careful titration, gradually adjusting the dose until the desired blood pressure is achieved, is vital for a safe and effective outcome.

Beyond the immediate actions, attention must be paid to maintaining normothermia. Hypothermia, a decrease in body temperature, can exacerbate hypotension by reducing cardiac output and peripheral vascular resistance. Keeping the patient warm, utilizing warming blankets or forced-air warming devices, can aid in blood pressure stabilization. This is particularly important in patients undergoing prolonged procedures or those who are already at risk for hypothermia due to pre-existing conditions or the anesthetic technique.

Postoperative monitoring of blood pressure is crucial, even after the procedure concludes. Patients should be closely observed for any signs of persistent hypotension or recurrence. A gradual return to baseline blood pressure is expected, but any significant deviation warrants prompt medical attention and a reassessment of fluid status and medication requirements. Early detection and prompt intervention are key to preventing serious complications and ensuring positive patient outcomes.

Prophylactic measures can also be implemented to minimize the risk of hypotension. These include optimizing the patient's hydration status preoperatively, addressing any pre-existing conditions that might increase the risk of hypotension, and selecting anesthetic agents with fewer hypotensive effects whenever possible. Furthermore, maintaining adequate blood volume throughout the procedure through careful fluid management can help prevent hypotension from developing. It's crucial to understand the individual patient's risk factors and adjust the approach accordingly. Each patient presents a unique set of circumstances, which influences the management strategy. This holistic approach highlights the importance of understanding the procedure, the patient, and the context.

A thorough understanding of the physiological mechanisms underlying hypotension, combined with skillful monitoring and appropriate treatment strategies, is essential for managing this potential complication effectively. The ability to recognize early warning signs and promptly intervene can significantly reduce the risks associated with hypotension, contributing to enhanced patient safety and a positive outcome for minimally invasive procedures. Remember, the primary goal is to maintain adequate tissue perfusion and prevent organ damage. Therefore, a proactive and individualized approach, tailored to each patient's specific needs and risks, is essential for successful hypotension management. The collaborative effort of the anesthesia team ensures that preventative measures and timely intervention are effectively implemented.

5.2 Respiratory Depression Management

Respiratory depression, a potentially life-threatening complication, necessitates immediate and effective intervention. Prompt recognition is crucial, relying on continuous monitoring of respiratory rate, depth, and effort. A decreased respiratory rate below 10 breaths per minute, shallow breathing, or the presence of apnea are all significant warning signs. Observe for signs of hypoxemia, such as cyanosis or altered mental status, further indicating the severity of the situation. Early detection significantly improves the chances of successful management and prevents serious sequelae.

The first step involves ensuring a patent airway. This may require simple maneuvers like repositioning the patient's head or suctioning any secretions obstructing the airway. If necessary, more advanced airway management techniques, such as insertion of an oropharyngeal or nasopharyngeal airway, or even endotracheal intubation, might become necessary. The choice of intervention will depend on the patient's clinical presentation and the available resources. Remember, maintaining

a clear airway is paramount in preventing further complications.
Oxygen supplementation is essential. Administering high-flow oxygen via a face mask or non-rebreather mask immediately increases oxygen saturation levels. Closely monitor oxygen saturation using pulse oximetry to assess the effectiveness of oxygen therapy and guide further interventions. Adequate oxygenation is critical in mitigating the effects of respiratory depression and preventing hypoxic tissue damage.
Pharmacological intervention often becomes necessary to reverse the effects of respiratory depressant drugs. Naloxone, a specific opioid antagonist, is used to counteract opioid-induced respiratory depression. Its administration should be guided by the patient's clinical response and continuous monitoring of vital signs. The dose may need to be titrated based on the individual's response, always prioritizing safety and observing for any potential adverse effects. In certain cases, other supportive medications might be required.
Maintaining adequate ventilation is another crucial element of effective management. If the patient's respiratory effort remains inadequate, despite the above measures, mechanical ventilation may be required. This could range from non-invasive ventilation with a CPAP or BiPAP machine to invasive mechanical ventilation with an endotracheal tube. The choice depends on the severity of the respiratory depression and the patient's overall clinical condition. Closely monitor ventilator settings and adjust them as needed to ensure adequate gas exchange and prevent complications associated with mechanical ventilation.
Post-intervention monitoring is as critical as immediate management. Continuously monitor respiratory rate, depth, and effort, along with oxygen saturation and vital signs. Assess the patient's level of consciousness and neurological status. The frequency of monitoring should be dictated by the patient's clinical stability, with more fre-

quent monitoring in unstable patients. Careful documentation of all interventions and responses is essential for effective communication and subsequent management. This allows for a complete picture of the patient's response to treatment and informs future decisions. Finally, remember that respiratory depression management is a collaborative effort. Effective communication and coordination among the anesthesia team, nursing staff, and other healthcare professionals are essential. Clear communication ensures everyone is informed about the patient's condition and the treatment plan, maximizing the effectiveness of care and ensuring the best possible outcome. Following established protocols and guidelines, while adapting to the specifics of each patient's situation, is crucial for safe and effective management. A thorough understanding of the underlying cause of respiratory depression can significantly influence treatment, promoting a personalized approach to ensure patient safety and well-being.

5.3 Allergic Reactions Management

Allergic reactions, while rare, represent a significant risk during minimally invasive procedures. Prompt recognition and treatment are paramount to ensuring patient safety. Understanding the potential allergens, recognizing symptoms, and implementing immediate interventions are crucial skills for any practitioner. This chapter provides a practical guide to managing these potentially life-threatening events. Immediate recognition of an allergic reaction is the first critical step. Symptoms can range from mild, such as localized itching or rash, to severe, including anaphylaxis, characterized by widespread hives, swelling of the face and throat (angioedema), respiratory distress, and cardiovascular collapse. The severity and speed of onset vary widely depending on the allergen, the dose received, and the individual patient's sensitivity. A detailed patient history, including known allergies, previous reactions, and any familial predisposition, is essential during the preoperative assessment. Remember, even seemingly mild allergies can become severe under the influence of other drugs or stresses.

For mild reactions, like localized itching or a mild rash, supportive measures often suffice. Discontinuing the suspected allergen is the first action. This might involve halting the infusion of a drug or removing a topical anesthetic. Oral antihistamines, such as diphenhydramine, can effectively manage symptoms such as itching and hives. Close observation for symptom progression is vital, as a seemingly minor reaction can escalate quickly. Documentation of the reaction, the interventions taken, and the patient's response is essential for both patient safety and legal reasons. Precise charting is key.

More severe reactions, however, require a much more aggressive approach. Anaphylaxis demands immediate, decisive intervention. This begins with securing the airway, which might involve inserting an endotracheal tube if respiratory distress is present. Administering oxygen is crucial, and supportive measures, such as intravenous fluids, may be necessary to maintain blood pressure. The cornerstone of anaphylaxis treatment is the prompt administration of epinephrine, which reverses the effects of histamine and other inflammatory mediators. Epinephrine should be given intramuscularly or intravenously, guided by established protocols and the severity of the reaction.

Beyond epinephrine, other medications may play a role in managing anaphylaxis. Intravenous fluids help maintain blood pressure and tissue perfusion. Broad-spectrum antihistamines, such as diphenhydramine or cetirizine, can further reduce symptoms and prevent further histamine release. Corticosteroids, such as methylprednisolone, are often given to reduce inflammation. Remember, these are supplementary treatments. Epinephrine is paramount. The treatment plan must be tailored to the specific presentation and severity of the reaction.

Post-reaction care is as crucial as immediate intervention. Continuous monitoring of vital signs is critical to detect any relapse or delayed reaction. Close observation for at least several hours is recommended. Patients experiencing severe anaphylactic reactions usually require close monitoring in a critical care setting, possibly needing further care in a hospital. Once the patient is stable, discharge planning must include detailed instructions on recognizing signs of recurrence and an action plan. This might involve educating the patient about carrying an epinephrine auto-injector. Finally, referral to an allergist for further testing and management of the allergy is vital to prevent future occurrences. Never underestimate the importance of communication with the patient and their family. They need to know how to recognize, understand, and address the allergy to prevent future complications.

6 Patient Selection and Preparation

A thorough patient history is paramount. We need to understand their medical background, including any allergies, current medications, and previous anesthetic experiences. This includes a detailed review of systems, focusing on cardiovascular, respiratory, and neurological health. Don't forget to inquire about family history of anesthetic complications, highlighting any potential genetic predispositions. Finally, a complete physical examination is vital, checking for any contraindications or potential risks. Detailed documentation is crucial for legal and continuity of care reasons.

Identifying the patient's level of anxiety regarding the procedure is key. Many individuals experience significant apprehension, and this fear can impact their physiological responses. Open communication is essential, allowing them to express their concerns. Addressing their anxieties head-on, providing reassurance, and answering their questions thoroughly helps build trust and improve their overall experience. Remember, a calm patient is a better patient.

Preoperative instructions need to be clear, concise, and tailored to the patient's individual needs and understanding. This includes detailed explanations of the procedure itself, the type of anesthesia or sedation being used, and potential side effects. We should provide specific instructions regarding food and drink restrictions, medication adjustments, and transportation arrangements. Written instructions, supplemented with visual aids where appropriate, are beneficial for reinforcing key information. Confirming the patient's understanding through their rephrasing of the instructions is critical.

Postoperative care plans are just as important as the preoperative preparation. This involves detailed instructions on pain management, including the use of prescribed analgesics, potential side effects to look out for, and when to seek immediate medical attention. We should also outline guidance on diet, activity restrictions, and wound care, where applicable. The frequency of follow-up appointments should be clearly communicated, along with contact information for immediate concerns. Individualized plans allow for seamless transitions from the procedural setting to recovery at home.

Establishing clear discharge criteria is essential for patient safety. This includes specific parameters related to vital signs, level of consciousness, pain control, and absence of complications. Patients should meet all criteria before being discharged. We must ensure they have a responsible adult accompanying them and that they understand the postoperative instructions thoroughly. Documenting the discharge process meticulously protects both the patient and the healthcare provider.

Patient education isn't a one-time event but an ongoing process. We should encourage patients to ask questions at any point and provide multiple avenues for clarification. This might include written materials, videos, or access to online resources, tailoring the information to meet their literacy level and comprehension capabilities. This comprehensive approach improves patient understanding, reduces anxiety, and fosters cooperation, leading to better outcomes. Providing easy-to-understand information promotes better patient compliance and overall satisfaction.

The selection and preparation of patients for minimally invasive procedures is a multi-faceted process. It demands attention to detail, individualization of care, and open communication. By focusing on patient history, managing anxiety, and providing clear instructions, we contribute to a safe and successful outcome, while promoting patient satisfaction and adherence to post-procedure care. Remember, thorough planning is the cornerstone of a positive experience for both the patient and healthcare professionals. A systematic approach minimizes risks and optimizes outcomes, aligning with ethical practices and ensuring the best possible patient care.

6.1 Patient History and Assessment

A comprehensive patient history is paramount. It's the cornerstone of a successful minimally invasive procedure, forming the basis for informed decisions regarding sedation and anesthesia choices. Gathering this information involves a detailed interview, carefully documenting the patient's medical background, current medications, allergies, and any relevant family history. This process helps identify potential risks and allows for personalized care planning, minimizing complications and ensuring patient safety. Understanding the patient's overall health status – including cardiovascular, respiratory, and neurological function – is crucial for risk stratification.

Thorough assessment extends beyond the medical history. A physical examination is equally important; it allows for a hands-on evaluation of the patient's condition, identifying any abnormalities that might influence the choice of anesthetic technique or necessitate modifications to the procedure itself. Assessing the patient's mental state is also critical; anxiety and fear can significantly impact a procedure's success, making a calm and reassuring approach essential. We should always validate their feelings and concerns. This holistic approach contributes significantly to the patient's overall well-being and procedural success.

The assessment needs to consider the specific procedure planned. Every intervention presents unique challenges and demands a tailored approach. For example, a minimally invasive dental procedure will have different considerations compared to a laparoscopic surgical intervention. Understanding the length, complexity, and potential risks of the procedure informs the selection of the most appropriate sedation and anesthesia method. This careful consideration minimizes potential side effects and ensures patient comfort. It also facilitates the efficient and effective use of resources, minimizing the overall time commitment for both patient and healthcare provider. Understanding the details of the procedure is integral to planning a safe and efficacious strategy.

Communication is key during both the history-taking and physical examination phases. Open dialogue with the patient builds trust and allows for a more accurate assessment. It ensures that the patient's concerns and preferences are addressed. Actively listening to the patient's narrative provides valuable insights into their perception of pain, anxiety levels, and previous experiences with medical interventions. This information may guide decisions regarding the type and level of sedation necessary to create a comfortable and safe environment. Remember, building trust is fundamental to a positive patient experience and successful procedure.

Beyond the immediate medical history, exploring the patient's lifestyle factors proves essential. Smoking, alcohol consumption, and drug use can significantly affect the body's response to anesthesia and sedation. These factors can increase the risks of complications and require careful consideration when choosing the anesthetic approach. It's equally important to gather information about the patient's diet and any underlying nutritional deficiencies that may influence their recovery process. A detailed understanding of the patient's lifestyle contributes to a complete clinical picture, which allows for more comprehensive and effective decision-making.

Finally, documenting all findings from the history and assessment is critical. A meticulously maintained record serves as a valuable resource for the entire care team. It aids in communication, reducing the risk of errors and ensuring continuity of care. This documentation also helps in tracking the patient's progress and evaluating the effectiveness of the chosen anesthetic method. Detailed records are vital for monitoring, evaluating the outcome and learning, particularly valuable in identifying any trends or patterns of complications that may inform future patient management strategies. Clear and comprehensive documentation represents a paramount aspect of safe and high-quality medical care.

6.2 Preoperative Instructions

Clear communication is paramount. Patients need to understand the procedure thoroughly, including the anesthesia plan, potential risks, and what to expect before, during, and after. This involves a clear explanation of the type of anesthesia, be it local, regional, or conscious sedation. Detailed instructions should cover the need for fasting, medication adjustments, and any necessary pre-procedure tests. This ensures a smooth process, minimizing anxiety and potential complications. Remember, a well-informed patient is a more cooperative patient, leading to a better overall outcome.

Nausea and vomiting are common concerns. Preoperative instructions should explicitly address strategies to minimize these post-procedure side effects. This might include specific dietary recommendations in the days leading up to the procedure, guidance on avoiding certain foods and beverages, and the potential for anti-emetic medication. Emphasizing the importance of following these instructions closely is crucial for patient comfort and a quicker recovery. Thorough communication regarding potential side effects allows patients to proactively manage expectations.

Hydration is key. Dehydration can negatively impact the procedure and recovery. Patients should be instructed to maintain adequate hydration in the 24 hours prior, avoiding excessive caffeine or alcohol intake. Specific guidance on fluid intake, such as the number of glasses of water to consume, can prove beneficial. This simple yet crucial step minimizes complications arising from dehydration, optimizing patient health.

Medication management requires careful attention. Patients should be instructed to inform the anesthesiologist about all medications they are currently taking, including over-the-counter drugs, herbal supplements, and vitamins. This is vital to avoid potential drug interactions that can affect the anesthetic plan, possibly delaying or even compromising the procedure. This detailed approach minimizes risk and promotes safety. Open communication ensures the appropriate course of action.

The importance of transportation cannot be overlooked. Patients should arrange for reliable transportation home after the procedure, especially if sedation is used. They should understand that their reflexes and judgment may be impaired, even with minimal sedation. This precaution safeguards patient safety during the post-procedure period, preventing possible accidents or injuries. The emphasis on safe travel practices demonstrates responsibility and patient advocacy.

Preoperative anxiety is a common occurrence. Patients should be informed about the support available to manage anxiety. This could involve relaxation techniques, guided imagery, or even pre-procedure counseling. Options for medication to alleviate anxiety should also be discussed if appropriate. Providing resources and support addresses a key concern, promoting overall well-being. The ability to feel supported can significantly impact a patient's experience.

A signed consent form is non-negotiable. Ensure the patient thoroughly understands the procedure, the anesthesia plan, and the potential risks and benefits before signing the consent form. Address any questions or concerns they may have, ensuring they are fully informed and comfortable proceeding. The process should be a collaborative discussion, not a mere formality. This highlights respect for patient autonomy and legal responsibilities.

Post-procedure instructions must be clearly explained. These instructions should cover details about pain management, dietary restrictions, activity limitations, and follow-up appointments. Providing written instructions, along with verbal explanations, will aid comprehension. The clarity of the information is key to successful recovery, avoiding confusion or potentially dangerous practices.

Finally, open communication fosters trust. Encourage patients to ask questions, express concerns, and maintain open communication with their medical team throughout the process. Creating a supportive environment reduces anxiety and facilitates a successful procedure. A comfortable and informed patient is far more likely to experience a positive outcome and a smoother recovery. A collaborative approach ultimately benefits everyone involved.

6.3 Postoperative Care

Postoperative care is paramount to a patient's successful recovery following a minimally invasive procedure. It's not simply about monitoring vital signs; it's about anticipating potential complications and providing individualized support to ensure a smooth transition back to normal activities. This requires a holistic approach, encompassing both physical and psychological aspects of recovery.

Careful monitoring of vital signs, including heart rate, blood pressure, respiratory rate, and oxygen saturation, remains crucial in the immediate postoperative period. Any deviations from established baseline readings should be promptly addressed, potentially requiring intervention to manage hypotension, respiratory depression, or other adverse events. The vigilance of the healthcare team, their experience and quick thinking, are essential.

Pain management is another cornerstone of effective postoperative care. While minimally invasive techniques inherently reduce postoperative pain, residual discomfort is often present and requires careful attention. Appropriate analgesics, administered via the most suitable route–oral, intravenous, or regional–should be prescribed, tailored to the individual patient's needs and tolerance. We should always consider the patient's pain rating and their own description of their discomfort.

Hydration and nutrition also play vital roles in recovery. Maintaining adequate fluid intake is crucial to prevent dehydration, especially with potential nausea or vomiting. Early mobilization, within the limits of the patient's physical condition, is highly encouraged to prevent complications such as thromboembolism. It's important to assess each patient individually, knowing that what works well for one person might not work for another.

Patient education is integral to a successful postoperative outcome. Clear and concise instructions regarding pain management, activity restrictions, diet, and potential complications should be provided before discharge. This empowers patients to actively participate in their recovery and facilitates early identification of any emerging problems. Their understanding of their condition significantly influences their willingness to comply with the recommendations given.

Discharge criteria should be clearly defined and meticulously followed. This involves careful assessment of the patient's pain levels, mobility, and overall well-being. Ensuring the patient has a reliable support system at home to assist with their care also helps to ensure a smoother transition. It's equally important to provide detailed and accessible contact information for follow-up appointments and emergency situations, making sure they feel comfortable reaching out if anything is amiss.

Psychological support shouldn't be overlooked. Anxiety and fear are common among patients recovering from procedures, even minimally invasive ones. Providing a supportive and reassuring environment can considerably enhance the patient's comfort and contribute to a faster and more comprehensive recovery. We must provide information and answer their questions openly and honestly, dispelling unfounded anxieties.

Finally, comprehensive documentation of all aspects of postoperative care is critical. This serves not only as a record of the patient's progress but also as a valuable tool for continuous improvement and quality assurance. It helps track the effectiveness of various interventions and aids in identifying areas where further improvement is needed. Through detailed records, we can learn from past practices and continually refine our approach to post-operative care.

6.4 Discharge Criteria

Safe discharge following minimally invasive procedures hinges on a comprehensive assessment encompassing several key factors. The patient's vital signs, including heart rate, blood pressure, respiratory rate, and oxygen saturation, must return to within acceptable ranges of their baseline or pre-procedure values. A stable level of consciousness, free from any lingering effects of sedation or anesthesia, is paramount. This means the patient is alert, oriented to person, place, and time, and can adequately respond to simple commands. Their ability to safely ambulate and maintain their balance without assistance, indicating adequate neurological function and minimizing the risk of falls, is also crucial. Furthermore, the absence of any significant pain, nausea, or vomiting should be confirmed, mitigating potential complications related to post-procedure discomfort or compromised hydration. The patient's ability to understand and retain discharge instructions are equally important.

Postoperative pain management should be addressed proactively. A plan for managing any anticipated discomfort should be in place before discharge, ensuring the patient has the necessary pain relief methods and understands how and when to use them. This includes providing clear instructions on pain medication, including dosage, frequency, and potential side effects. Adequate pain control is essential to enable the patient to resume normal activities and prevent potential complications associated with uncontrolled pain. The importance of this cannot be overstated, as effective pain management significantly contributes to a smoother recovery and a positive patient experience. Therefore, a comprehensive discharge plan includes a detailed explanation of potential side effects, the importance of adherence to the prescribed medication regimen, and when to seek additional medical attention.

The patient's understanding of the procedure, any potential complications, and recovery expectations plays a crucial role in successful discharge. A clear explanation of potential side effects, including their severity and likelihood, is essential, ensuring informed consent and empowering the patient. This also includes providing contact information for follow-up appointments or for emergencies. Clear communication enhances patient understanding and reduces anxiety which leads to a smoother transition back to their regular lives. The discussion should also cover potential complications, emphasizing the need to seek immediate medical attention if any arise. Providing written instructions reinforces the verbal explanation, helping ensure that the patient has a clear understanding of all instructions before leaving the care facility.

Beyond the immediate physical state, the social and psychological aspects of the patient's readiness for discharge also warrant consideration. Support systems, such as family members or caregivers, should be assessed to ensure adequate assistance is available during the initial recovery period at home. This includes verifying the availability of someone to help the patient with tasks like medication administration, transportation, or meal preparation, especially if mobility or dexterity is limited. Addressing emotional support and any concerns that the patient might have is integral to this stage. Ensuring that the patient feels confident in their ability to manage their recovery effectively helps prevent potential complications and promotes a positive patient experience. A comprehensive evaluation of the patient's emotional state, understanding, and available support is vital for determining their readiness for discharge.

Finally, the patient's home environment should be assessed for suitability. Any potential hazards in the home environment must be identified and addressed to minimize risks. This could include addressing tripping hazards, ensuring appropriate lighting, and confirming the availability of essential supplies like medications and medical equipment. Patients should be reassured that they can contact the medical team if they experience any issues following discharge. By addressing these factors, we can significantly enhance patient safety, facilitate recovery, and optimize the overall discharge process, making the transition back to a normal life as comfortable and efficient as possible. A safe discharge contributes to a positive patient experience and reinforces confidence in the benefits of minimally invasive procedures.

6.5 Patient Education

Effective patient education is paramount for successful minimally invasive procedures. It fosters trust, reduces anxiety, and ensures patients actively participate in their care, leading to better outcomes and improved satisfaction. This contributes to a positive patient experience and enhances the overall effectiveness of the procedure. A well-informed patient is better equipped to manage expectations and adhere to post-procedural instructions, contributing to faster recovery and fewer complications.

Preparing patients begins with a clear and concise explanation of the procedure itself. Use simple, non-medical terms to describe the process, the anticipated sensations, and the duration of the procedure. Visual aids, such as diagrams or videos, can greatly enhance understanding, particularly for complex procedures. Remember to check for comprehension at every step and offer the opportunity for questions, even if they seem trivial.

Addressing patient anxieties is equally crucial. Many patients experience fear of needles, pain, or complications. Openly acknowledging these concerns and validating their feelings creates a safe space for communication. Emphasize the advantages of minimally invasive techniques–reduced pain, faster recovery, and a shorter hospital stay–while honestly discussing potential risks and complications, however unlikely. Providing realistic expectations significantly contributes to anxiety reduction.

Detailed instructions for pre-operative preparation must be provided. This includes dietary restrictions, medication adjustments, and any required pre-procedure tests or assessments. Provide written instructions to complement the verbal explanation, reinforcing key information and offering a lasting reference for the patient. Clearly state any necessary fasting periods and explain why they are essential for safety. Provide contact information for questions and concerns before the procedure, reassuring patients they are not alone in the preparation process.

Post-operative care instructions require equal attention. Discuss potential side effects, including pain management strategies, wound care guidelines, and any activity restrictions. Explain the importance of follow-up appointments and provide contact information in case of unexpected complications. It's important to ensure the patient understands the signs and symptoms that need immediate attention, empowering them to take proactive steps to manage their recovery. Offering clear, concise, and easily understood instructions helps to ensure that patients follow them precisely, leading to quicker recoveries.

Effective communication goes beyond just providing information. It's about actively listening to the patient's concerns, addressing their questions with empathy, and tailoring the educational approach to their individual needs and learning styles. Building rapport with the patient will result in a more collaborative and trusting relationship, thereby improving outcomes and increasing patient satisfaction. Remember that open communication leads to improved patient compliance, reduced anxiety, and ultimately, a better post-procedure experience.

Tailoring the information to the patient's specific literacy level and cultural background is vital. Use simple language and avoid medical jargon. For those with limited health literacy, consider using visual aids or even employing a family member or translator to ensure complete comprehension. Consider the patient's educational level and any cultural beliefs that may influence their understanding and acceptance of the procedure. A multi-faceted approach which includes visual tools and simplified language will ensure better engagement and understanding across diverse patient demographics.

Finally, actively soliciting feedback from the patient is essential. Ask them to summarize the information to gauge their understanding and identify any areas requiring clarification. Encouraging questions and creating a judgement-free environment will support patient comprehension and improve the overall effectiveness of the patient education process. Following the procedure, obtain feedback on their experience and the clarity of the instructions provided to ensure continuous improvement. Remember that the ultimate goal is to empower patients to be active participants in their own care, fostering a positive and successful outcome.

7 Future Trends in Minimally Invasive Anesthesia

The field of minimally invasive anesthesia is constantly evolving, driven by the pursuit of enhanced patient comfort and safety. We are witnessing a surge in technological advancements that promise to redefine the landscape of procedural sedation and analgesia. One exciting area lies in the development of sophisticated sedation devices that offer greater precision and control. These devices often incorporate closed-loop systems, dynamically adjusting medication delivery based on real-time patient physiological data. This results in a more tailored and responsive approach to sedation management, minimizing the risk of both under\item and over-sedation.

Imagine a future where administering anesthesia becomes less reliant on subjective assessment and more guided by objective, quantifiable data. This is the promise of advanced monitoring systems that integrate various physiological parameters and predictive algorithms to optimize anesthesia delivery. Such integrated systems could analyze multiple data points - heart rate variability, respiratory patterns, even subtle changes in brainwave activity - providing clinicians with a more comprehensive picture of the patient's response to anesthesia.

Beyond sophisticated devices, research is actively exploring novel anesthetic agents with improved safety profiles and faster recovery times. These agents might offer a greater therapeutic index, allowing for more precise dosing and reduced side effects. Some promising avenues include targeted drug delivery systems, designed to concentrate the anesthetic in the desired area, minimizing systemic exposure and side effects. The development of biodegradable and biocompatible materials for local anesthetic delivery systems also represents a significant advancement, potentially eliminating the need for invasive injections.

The incorporation of advanced imaging technologies, such as ultrasound and near-infrared spectroscopy, is another significant trend. These technologies allow for real-time visualization of anatomical structures and tissue perfusion, improving the accuracy of nerve blocks and regional anesthesia techniques. Moreover, continuous monitoring of tissue oxygenation can further minimize complications and ensure adequate tissue perfusion during procedures. This level of visualization and monitoring significantly reduces the risk of complications associated with traditional blind techniques.

Furthermore, the integration of artificial intelligence and machine learning algorithms is poised to revolutionize anesthesia delivery. AI-powered systems could analyze vast datasets of patient information, including medical history, physiological parameters, and procedural details, to predict individual responses to anesthesia. This allows for personalized anesthesia protocols and a proactive approach to managing potential complications. The potential for AI to enhance the accuracy and efficiency of anesthesia delivery is immense, promising improved patient outcomes and a more streamlined workflow for healthcare providers.

The integration of virtual reality (VR) and augmented reality (AR) technologies in procedural sedation represents another exciting development. VR can help patients relax and reduce anxiety before and during procedures, potentially decreasing the need for deeper sedation. AR can provide clinicians with real-time, interactive overlays on anatomical imaging, enhancing their ability to perform minimally invasive procedures. By creating a more immersive and distraction-free experience for patients, these technologies could contribute to a more comfortable and efficient procedural environment.

Looking further into the future, there's considerable research exploring the use of targeted gene therapy and other innovative techniques for pain management. While still in the early stages, these approaches might eventually offer long-lasting pain relief, drastically reducing or eliminating the need for repeated anesthetic interventions. Such developments could significantly impact the management of chronic pain conditions, improving the overall quality of life for millions of individuals. Early indications are promising, suggesting new approaches to pain management are on the horizon.

However, as we advance into this era of innovative anesthesia techniques, it's crucial to remain mindful of ethical considerations and patient safety. The responsible implementation of these technologies requires rigorous clinical trials, careful monitoring, and robust quality assurance measures. Open communication between healthcare providers and patients remains paramount, fostering mutual understanding and ensuring informed consent. The responsible integration of these technological advances is critical to realize the full potential of minimally invasive anesthesia while maintaining the highest standards of patient care. The goal, ultimately, is to provide safe, effective, and personalized anesthesia care that enhances patient comfort and well-being. The ongoing evolution of minimally invasive anesthesia techniques is a testament to this unwavering dedication.

7.1 Advanced Sedation Devices

Precise delivery of sedative agents is paramount for successful minimally invasive procedures. Advanced sedation devices offer significant improvements over traditional methods, minimizing the risk of complications and enhancing patient comfort. These devices often incorporate sophisticated monitoring capabilities, providing real-time feedback on the patient's physiological response to the sedative. This allows for a more tailored and precise approach to sedation management, ensuring the optimal level of sedation is achieved and maintained throughout the procedure.

Target-controlled infusion (TCI) pumps represent a significant advancement. They allow for the precise delivery of sedatives based on the desired plasma concentration, rather than relying on fixed infusion rates. This allows for greater control over the depth and duration of sedation, reducing the risk of over-sedation or under-sedation. TCI pumps require careful calibration and programming, understanding the pharmacokinetic and pharmacodynamic parameters of the chosen sedative. Clinicians need to account for individual patient variations in metabolism and drug clearance for successful TCI administration. This level of precise control offers a remarkable advantage compared to traditional methods of manual bolus administration.

Another area of significant advancement lies in the development of sophisticated monitoring systems integrated with sedation delivery devices. These systems often include features like pulse oximetry, capnography, and electrocardiography, providing a comprehensive view of the patient's physiological status. Real-time data visualization allows for immediate detection of subtle changes, indicating potential complications like respiratory depression or hypotension. Early detection is crucial, as prompt intervention can prevent the escalation of adverse events. The incorporation of alarm systems into these devices is a noteworthy safety feature, automatically alerting the clinician to critical changes.

Beyond TCI pumps, closed-loop sedation systems are emerging. These systems use advanced algorithms to dynamically adjust the rate of sedative delivery in response to real-time patient data. For instance, the system might automatically reduce the infusion rate if the patient's respiratory rate falls below a predetermined threshold, thus preventing respiratory depression. This level of automation offers the potential for improved safety and efficiency compared to traditional methods that rely on the clinician's judgment alone. This level of automation and integration improves safety and efficiency but requires thorough training and appropriate clinical governance to ensure safe deployment.

The integration of artificial intelligence and machine learning into sedation devices also holds promise. These technologies could be used to predict individual patient responses to sedation, allowing for more personalized dosing strategies. This approach could further reduce the risk of complications, thereby enhancing the overall safety and efficacy of minimally invasive procedures. However, it's critical that these technological advancements be deployed responsibly, considering the potential biases that may exist within AI algorithms and that thorough validation and testing are completed before widespread use.

However, the use of advanced sedation devices is not without challenges. The cost associated with these devices can be substantial, posing a barrier to their widespread adoption, particularly in resource-constrained settings. Furthermore, these devices may require more extensive training and expertise to operate effectively, demanding further investment in training and education for healthcare professionals. This necessitates thoughtful implementation strategies considering both financial feasibility and professional development needs.

In conclusion, advanced sedation devices represent a significant advancement in the field of minimally invasive anesthesia and sedation. They offer several advantages including improved precision in drug delivery, enhanced monitoring capabilities, and the potential for automated responses to patient changes. While challenges remain regarding cost and training requirements, the potential benefits in terms of patient safety and comfort warrant further investigation and adoption of these innovative technologies. The future of minimally invasive procedures will likely see these devices becoming even more sophisticated and integrated, leading to even safer and more effective sedation practices. As technology continues to evolve, the focus should remain on the ethical considerations and equitable access to these advancements, ensuring that all patients benefit from these improvements. This necessitates ongoing collaboration between researchers, clinicians, and regulatory bodies to ensure responsible development and implementation.

7.2 New Anesthesia Techniques

The development of new anesthetic agents continues to revolutionize minimally invasive procedures. We're seeing a shift towards agents with faster onsets and shorter durations of action, minimizing recovery times and improving patient comfort. For instance, dexmedetomidine, an alpha-2 adrenergic agonist, offers unique advantages in providing both sedation and analgesia, reducing the need for multiple drugs. Its shorter half-life compared to traditional agents like propofol allows for more precise control and a quicker return to baseline function. This targeted approach minimizes the risks associated with prolonged sedation, enhancing patient safety and satisfaction.

Research into novel anesthetic delivery methods is also yielding exciting results. Targeted drug delivery systems, such as liposomal or nanoparticle-based formulations, offer the potential for increased efficacy with reduced side effects. Imagine delivering an anesthetic agent directly to the target nerve or tissue, eliminating systemic effects. This could revolutionize regional anesthesia, drastically minimizing complications and maximizing patient comfort. These targeted delivery systems require sophisticated infrastructure and specialized training, but their potential benefits warrant further investment and research.

Beyond the chemical advancements, the integration of advanced imaging techniques with anesthesia administration shows remarkable promise. Real-time ultrasound guidance for nerve blocks, for example, allows for more precise needle placement and reduces the risk of complications such as nerve injury. This improved precision not only enhances the effectiveness of the block but also significantly improves the patient experience. Similar advancements are occurring with computer-aided imaging for regional anesthesia, guiding practitioners in real time and minimizing invasiveness.

Furthermore, the field of personalized anesthesia is emerging. Genetic testing may one day allow us to tailor anesthetic regimens to individual patient needs, minimizing risks and optimizing therapeutic effects. This approach, while still in its early stages, has the potential to significantly improve patient outcomes. Imagine predicting a patient's susceptibility to complications based on their genetic profile, allowing for preemptive interventions and preventative care. The ethical considerations of such personalized approaches need careful consideration, alongside the potential legal liabilities and requirements for detailed documentation of patient genetic data.

Combining established techniques with innovative approaches is vital. For example, the use of ultrasound-guided nerve blocks in conjunction with local anesthetic infiltration can optimize analgesic effects.

Combining these approaches, and tailoring anesthetic strategy to individual patients based on pre-operative assessment, can allow for significantly shorter procedure times, with a corresponding decrease in overall anesthesia time and reduced risk of complications. The synergy between techniques is key for optimal pain management, reduced recovery time, and greater patient safety.

The future of anesthesia holds incredible potential. By continually embracing new technologies and refining existing techniques, we can create a safer, more effective, and more comfortable experience for patients undergoing minimally invasive procedures. This continued focus on innovation, coupled with meticulous patient selection, rigorous monitoring, and a thorough understanding of potential complications, represents our collective commitment to providing the highest quality of care. Ongoing commitment to research and education is essential to ensure the safe and effective implementation of these advancements. This includes not just mastering the techniques but also navigating the ethical and logistical challenges posed by these new technologies. The pursuit of painless procedures requires a collaborative effort between researchers, clinicians, and industry professionals, resulting in better patient outcomes and enhanced healthcare standards.

www.ingramcontent.com/pod-product-compliance
Lightning Source LLC
LaVergne TN
LVHW022023200926
848481LV00007B/2512
9798349295492